SIMPLE BODY DETOX METHOD

SIMPLE BODY
DETOX METHOD

SPECIAL SECRET RESOURCE!

Detox Your Body... And Your Life!

Frustrated With Yourself For Letting All The Toxins Eat Your Body Out? Still Confused As To How To Get Rid Of Them? Don't Know Where And How To Start? Fret Not, There Is Light At The End Of The Tunnel!

At Last! A Powerful Info-packed Guide That Has Some Of The Never-seen-before Tips And Tricks That Would Help You Get Rid Of The Toxins In Your Body! You Can Instantly Start The Detoxification Process And Save Your Body From Corrosion...!

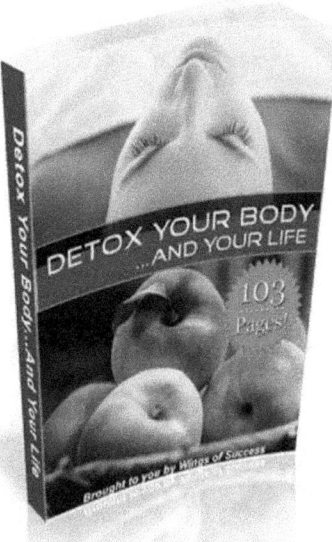

AVAILABLE ONLY FOR A VERY LIMITED TIME!

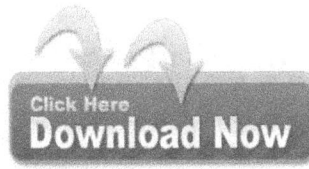
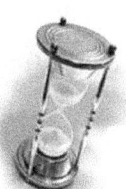

Body Detox Made Easy!

Master Cleanse Secrets

Curious About The Master Cleanse? Then You Need To Know...

The Master Cleanse Is Not As Easy As Everyone Thinks - Here's How You Can Avoid The Side Effects And Comfortably Finish The Master Cleanse

10 Days To A Whole New You

- ✓ You'll normalize your appetite and metabolism so your body can comfortably adjust to it's ideal weight for your size naturally
- ✓ Your suppressed hormone levels will be restored so every cell in your body will be charged with youth giving and feel good hormones
- ✓ There will be a natural shift away from unhealthy habits--without will power
- ✓ You'll cleanse and detox your entire body--the pounds of waste built up over the years will be released in just 10 days
- ✓ Reduced internal inflammation, which will ease aching joints
- ✓ Your energy levels will sore
- ✓ And much more...

Pounds Of Putrid Waste Eliminated For Good

DOWNLOAD NOW

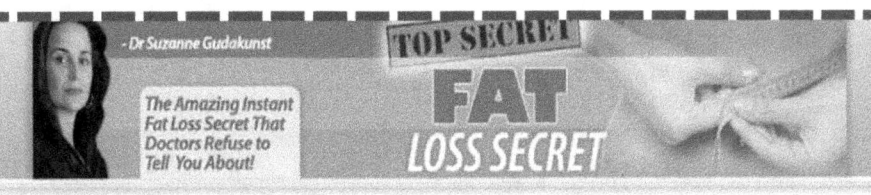

World-Famous TV Lady Doctor comes forth and blows the lid off the conspiracy to keep you unhealthy, fat & just plain sick...

Shocking Proof!

Here's the real reason you're fat...

"The Reason You Can't Lose Weight has Nothing to Do With Your *Will-Power*, *Over-Eating* or the *Right Diet!* ... The Reason You are Fat and Unhealthy is Because You Have Disgusting *Plaque* and Horrible Little 'CRITTERS' Living in Your Guts!"

"...And Now I'm Going to Show You How to Get Rid of All of It so You Can Shed 10 lbs, 25 lbs, 50 lbs even 100 lbs or more - and Keep It Off FOREVER!!"

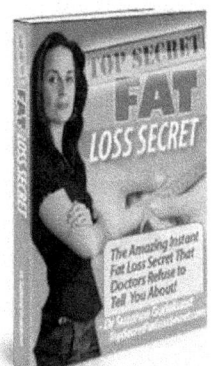

TOP SECRET
Fat Loss Secret

DOWNLOAD NOW

SIMPLE BODY DETOX METHOD

Body Detox Made Easy!

Contents

A 10-Day Body Detox..................8
Keep A Body Detox Journal..................10
Body Detox For Better Skin..................12
Body Detox Products – An Easy Way To Detoxify Your Self..................13
Detox- Cleansing the Body Inside Out..................15
Detox Home Kit: Easier Way of Improving Your Body..................17
Body Detox Herbs Can Do Wonder in Your Lives..................19
Detox through Tao for a Natural Way to Purify the Body for Health..................21
Detox Diets 101: Keeping Your body in Shape through Proper eating..................23
All natural body detox for body cleansing and total mind rejuvenation..................25
When to Say That Detox Diet Guide on Cleansing Your Body Is Safe..................27
A rejuvenating 5-day body detox plan to keep you going..................29
Gentler Ways to Detox the Body..................31
Balancing Ph-ion and Detox to Cleanse the Body..................33
Cleanse Yourself and do Body Detox for better Health..................35
Body Detox: The Process to Purify Your Life, Mind, and Soul..................38
Healthy Eating with Detox Recipes for your Body..................41
Home Body-Detox Programs for Losing Weight..................43
Detox Body in 7 Days with Internal Cleansers..................46
Body Detox- The Elemis Silhouette Body Contouring Capsule..................48
Body Detox the Easy Way: A Natural Diet..................50
Detox- The Natural Way..................52
Detox- Why it is necessary..................54
Detox foot patch..................56
How Detox Wrap Works Miracles to Your Body..................58
Detox- For the mind, body and Spirit..................60
Detox- Bruce Fife tells you how..................62
Using natural herbs for Detox..................64
Procedures For Natural Body Detox..................66

A 10-Day Body Detox

Are you looking for a full total body detox? If so, then you might want to try a 10 day detox or some refer to it as the 2-week detox. A 10-day detox is a full body detox that usually means taking several different steps to reach your total body transformation. It might involve a change in diet, exercise and more.

A full body detox is more thorough than a 24-hour fast of 72-hour juice diet. You need a full body detox program and you need to be ready to commit the full amount of time that it will take to get the full benefit of your detox.

You need a system that can help you by:

o   Removing heavy metals such as lead and mercury
o   Detoxify your liver, kidneys and other organs – even the brain
o   Replenish the friendly bacteria with a pro-biotic formula
o   Recharge your immune system with a powerful antioxidant support

You might also want to work on your emotional state and detoxing your mind. While your brain is an organ as well and will get the same benefit from detoxing the other organs of your body, detoxing the soul is a bit different.

If you want to cleanse and refresh your body, it is a great idea to cleanse and refresh your mind and spirit at the same time which can be done in a 10-day full body detox. Spend time relaxing, recouping and retraining your mind. Take time to de-stress from all the worries and trouble in the world and in your life while also cleansing your body physically.

You might want to try journaling and breathing and relaxing exercises in addition to the ingested regimen you have for your 10 day detox. You will come out of the process feeling like a new person.

What Is A Body Detox Routine?

Are you planning a body detox to cleanse your body? If you want to try a body detox either for your first time or if you have done it before, you will want to have a detox routine. So what exactly is a detox routine? Basically a detox routine is an all-natural method of cleansing your body by giving it the time and conditions it needs to rebuild and heal from the damages of daily life and the foods you eat and other substances you intake.

There are many different types of known detox routines. Some common types include:
o juicefasting
o waterfasting
o minimaleating/fasting
o herbaldetoxification
o detoxbaths
o coloncleansing
o caloricrestriction
o andmanymore

Your detox routine will be the specific plan that you take to detoxify and rejuvenate your body. It might be a pre-purchased plan that you get which contains all the steps needed for a healthy detox or it might be a plan that you helped formulate yourself.

You might want to try different detox routines or different combinations of different detoxification routines until you find one that works well for you. Once you find something that works well for you, you can continue to use it every time your body needs a detox.

How often you detox will also depend on your routine, the type of routine you use and how often you plan to use it. It will vary according to what your regular lifestyle is as well. After your detox, do you continue to eat healthy and avoid things that create a lot of toxins? If so, then you will not need your detox routine very often.

If you detox and then go back to a poor diet, caffeine and sugar and even nicotine, then you will need another detox sooner as your body will have more build up of toxins faster.

Keep A Body Detox Journal

If you are going to perform a body detox, you should keep a detox journal along the way to help you. You can get any kind of notebook, binder, paper, etc to write on and something comfortable to write with and begin making notes from day one. Your journal can look anyway you want or be any type of book that you want and you feel comfortable with. The point is just to keep notes on your life and your experiences during the detox.

You might write down the steps that you take in your detox, what you consume, what you restrict, etc. You might also write down your feelings and emotions along the way as well. Write anything and everything that you want while you are going through the detox program even if it does not directly apply to your detox. Just your emotions and state of mind at this point can be very insightful to read later.

Benefits of A Body Detox Journal

There are actually many different benefits to keeping your detox journal. For one, you can write down all of the steps you take and what you experience along the way. This will help you remember how to do things the next time you detox and if something does not work well for you, you will know how to change it next time. You can compare your detox experiences over the years and see how they change and how you grow as a person.

Another reason why it is a good idea is because many people experience mood swings and other moodiness while going through a detoxification. This lets you write down how you feel and helps you sort through your moods and emotions. It also helps you grow emotionally and you can look back on your journals later.

Body Detox For Your Mind

You hear all of this talk about body detox and what it can do for your health. You probably understand what it can do for your body but do you know what it can do for your mind?

If you want to detox your mind, you will want to create a "cleansing day". Because life brings many stresses and worries from day to day, you will want to have a regular cleansing day not just one time and then never again. You might want to detox your mind once a week or once every two weeks. If you are really pushed for time, you might go longer than that but the more often, the better so your mind doesn't get clogged down again.

One way you can release many of your past stresses, worries and fears is to keep a journal to write daily about how you feel. Or maybe if you don't have time to write daily you can write only on your cleansing day. You might also want to write letters (that you don't send) to yourself or friends or family members writing about your emotions, events that happened and other things to help you release stress that clogs up the mind.

You need to be careful not to try to just push away negative feelings. They never truly disappear and they just get clogged in your system and come back later bigger to make you feel worse of they lie there quietly but nag at you little by little with each passing day. Instead, take these feeling and embrace them but move on as a smarter person and don't hold to past pains and regrets.

These are great steps to take to detoxify the mind and start living a new fresh life with less worries and fears. A detox of the mind will also help you feel better and healthier as a person.

Body Detox For Better Skin

You might have heard about body detox and all the great things it can do for you. You probably have also heard that it can help cleanse your colon, remove toxins and waste from the body and help prevent disease and illness. You probably also know that it can give you more energy and boost your immune system.

Did you know that a body detox can also give you great skin? If you want to have younger, smoother, healthier looking skin, then a detoxification of your body might be the way to go. It can make your skin look and feel refreshed. By cleaning out the toxins in your body, the result is that you look and feel healthier all over. Our skin is often a sign of our inner health. People that are unhealthy may have dry, brittle skin, more wrinkles and more signs of age than a healthier person.

Toxins in the body can cause your skin to be pale and dry and look unhealthy. It can contribute to signs of aging earlier as well. When you clean your body deeply from the inside out, you remove these toxins that weigh down on your body and skin and refresh yourself. In the days that follow your detoxification, you should notice your skin becoming healthier and more alive. Over time, this will continue. Drinking a lot of water- whether it was specified in your detox program or not- will also be very helpful.

There are also special skin detox formulas you can purchase that are specifically for people with problem skin, acne or other skin conditions. There are many specially formulated detox systems that are designed for people that have skin problems or for those that might be experiencing aging and fine lines or wrinkles and just want to rejuvenate their skin.

Body Detox Products – An Easy Way To Detoxify Your Self

No one is a 100 percent free of toxins inside. I mean that the detoxification process is not always a hundred percent successful and the body needs some external help with the detoxification process. This can be achieved in many ways including dieting, use of detox kits and other medication especially herbal detoxification tonics and pills.

People are of the belief that they are free of toxins because they are in total control of the cleanliness. Nothing can be further from the truth. There are toxins in everything we consume, and when we are not consuming it is entering our system through the pores of our skin and he air we breathe. The vegetables we eat are sprayed with pesticides which are not completely washed off before cooking. These chemicals turn up in our system as toxins.

The air we breathe is polluted with smoke and petroleum fumes, in addition to this there are chemicals in the house that come from the toiletries we use. These sprays and shampoos and soaps are loaded with toxins that will enter our system through our eyes, nose and skin and later build up to such an extent that it will be almost impossible for the natural process of the body to rid itself of them. Toxins in the body will eventually lead to health problems and so must be purged from the body at regular intervals to prevent a build up of toxin levels.

Medical science has come a long way and with it comes many discoveries in the detoxification process of he human body. Humans have developed ways to increase their life span and treat symptoms of dreaded diseases and alleviate a lot of pain through proper medical procedures. However, it is these same medications that leave behind a residue that builds up as toxins in the system. These toxins have their own side effects. In fact any kind of medication adds to the build up of toxins in the system. It is imperative that these toxins should be purged from the system to prevent any health problems in time.

Our kidney and liver are able to rid the system of toxins to a great extent, however, when the toxins build up to such an extent it is important for us to find the right detox product to help the process along. There are detox kits that can be used in he home and they do a very good job too. These kits contain detox herbal products that can be used along with a diet plan that comes with the detox kit. In about 5 days you will be relatively free from toxins in your body with proper use of these detox products. It is equally important to find the right detox product that works well for you. This could mean a bit of trial and error but before long you will definitely find it.

Detox- Cleansing The Body Inside Out

It is important to cleanse the body of the toxins that have accumulated through the months. These toxins play havoc with the vital organs of the body and leave a trail of destruction. They need to be removed from the system without trace – if that were possible.

In order to cleanse the system of toxins one must clean the colon. It is said that death begins with the malfunction of the colon. Though the kidneys and the liver are primarily responsible for the cleansing of toxins from the system the colon is a vital player in assisting the process of detoxification. So where do these toxins come from? There are many sources for toxins that enter the body through every possible opening, including the tiny pores in the skin.

The air we breathe is a rich source of toxins that make their way into our blood stream. Toxins are deposited into the air through car fumes and pollution from industries. The vegetables we eat are polluted with toxins through the insecticides we spray to kill the pests that destroy the plants. The chemical fertilizer we use for the plants is another source of toxins that make their way into the vegetables and fruit we eat. The water we drink is treated with cleansing and purification agents, again chemicals. These make their way into our system and finally add to the toxic levels in our body.

Another great source of toxins is the medications that we take to heal ourselves. In fact, any form of chemical intake leads to the build up of toxins in out system. Then again here are the chemical toiletries such as deodorants and sprays; these are a big source of toxins.

So, how do toxins affect our system?
Toxins affect all the organs of our body. They mainly attack the kidneys, liver and the colon. Toxins hamper the functioning of the immune system and leave the body open to attacks from diseases leading to ill health. Some of the main symptoms are aging, skin rashes and many other skin disorders, indigestion, nausea, and most of all behavioral changes including depression, a rising disorder linked to toxin levels in the system.

The best way to rid the system of toxins is to go on a detox diet. This is a program that consists on vegetables and fruits. A 5 day diet of leafy vegetables and fresh fruit along with at least 4 liters of water every day will rid the system of over 80% toxins. There are other ways that include home detox kits complete with herbal detox pills and tonics that work independently on each organ to detoxify the system.

Whatever the process you choose to detoxify your body it is important to do so on a regular basis such as twice a year. A detoxified body is a healthy body and a happier individual.

Detox Home Kit: Easier Way Of Improving Your Body

The market is agog with detox products. These products come in the form of kits that consist of written detox diet plans and accompanied by herbal pills and tonics that are used to cleanse the system of toxins. There are different herbs that must be taken together to cleanse or detoxify the different organs of the body simultaneously to achieve complete detoxification of the system.

However, one should bear in mind that these herbal detox products have no scientific testing procedure or evidence to prove hat they actually detoxify the system of harmful chemicals and toxins. This is proven by the fact that the manufacturers of the herbal detox products do not publish any evidence of the efficiency of the system, they just rely on the testimonials of the people who have used the herbal products and are satisfied with the results.

According to the testimonials the detox kits are very effective in cleaning the system of toxins that have accumulated over the years. The cleansing process rejuvenates the mind and body allowing it to function more effectively leaving he person with a feeling of well being. Many people are of the view that fasting is a good way to cleanse the system of toxins; detoxification is a much more effective way to achieve better results. Herbal detox kits flush out the toxins from the body and keep them out to a great extent.

The build up of the toxin levels in the system may cause many diseases including degenerative diseases the main ones being accelerated aging of a person with high levels of toxins. Toxins may bring out any emotional trauma that has been suppressed for many years causing complications and ill health. Some of the symptoms of toxification are indigestion, nausea and liver disease. If you are aware of any of these symptoms you should be on the look out for changes in your behavior as well. A high level of toxins in the body will lead to mood swings and depression in extreme cases. If you ignore these symptoms you will be inviting nothing but trouble.

Though it is impossible to prevent exposure to toxins in today's day and age it is important to learn how to control the toxification of the system. This will help us to lead a healthier life style. By preventing ourselves to unnecessary exposure of toxins the body has to face difficulty in purging them. These toxins can ultimately accumulate and cause problems for us. Detox kits are a great way to detoxify our systems and prevent any unnecessary health problems.

These home kits effectively remove toxins over a period of 5 days without any side effects and can be used at least twice a year to maintain a healthy system.

Body Detox Herbs Can Do Wonder In Your Lives

It is a well known fact that the atmosphere and the food we eat and drink are crammed with harmful chemicals that enter the body and add to the build up of toxins that hamper the proper functioning of the body. Add to this the pesticides and fumes we breathe in unknowingly adding to the build up of toxins. Before long the body will begin to reel under the effects of these harmful toxins and will need to be cleansed. This cleansing process is called detoxification.

Our body does have a natural cleansing mechanism and this works through the kidney and liver at times the system can become over burdened and may need some external help from us to clean out the circulatory and excretory systems of the body. Some of the processes practiced for detoxification is prolonged fasting. This is an unhealthy process as the body needs nutrients to sustain itself. The best way is to resort to a detox diet assisted with detox body herbs as well.

Since the immune system is the mechanism that defends he body from disease, toxins cause the person to fall ill as the immune system is the first to be affected by harmful levels of toxins in the system. This is why it is necessary to remove the toxins from the body through a detox process. The benefits of detox herbs is not unknown to the medical fraternity as a potent way to detoxify the system. These are the best and the most natural way to detoxify the system and instill a feeling of well being.

Some of the detoxifying herbs used to cleanse the system are:

1. **Psyllium seeds**. These herbs induce bowel movements and clean the bowls of toxins very effectively. The herb itself acts like a sponge absorbing the toxins and passing out with the excreta.

2. **Cascara Sagrada** is another very effective laxative that is used to flush out the toxins from the system and is used along with the psyllium seeds.

3. **Milk Thistle** simulates the protein synthesis in the liver the cleansing organ of the blood.

4. **Nettles** are used in combination with other detox herbs for cleaning the urinary system of toxins.

5. **Burdock roots** are used when the need to cleanse he system is very urgent. This herb reduces the build up of metals causing problems within the system.

6. **Dandelion roots** are herbs with the strongest detoxifying properties. These herbs are used to clean the gall bladder of waste as also the kidneys. The Dandelion root is used in conjunction with other detox herbs as other organs need to be cleansed simultaneously.

The main source of toxins for humans is the pollution in the air and the toxins present in the processed food we eat. Due to a lack of time people are turning more and more to processed foods not realizing the health hazard they are exposing themselves to. Toxins need to be purged from the system and many people are doing this twice a year. Doctors emphasize that the need to detoxify our system is indeed necessary, however, the more natural the process the better it will be.

Detox Through Tao For A Natural Way To Purify The Body For Health

Many people feel very safe in their homes and offices. They feel that they can control the level of cleanliness and pollution in their familiar surroundings; however, it is time to give some serious thought to this once and for all. The water we drink and the food we eat as well as the air we breathe are all full of toxins that add up in our systems and finally make our vital organs malfunction.

The world is not what our ancestors or even our grand parents knew it. In their time the world and its environment was a different, cleaner and safer place to live. Pollution is a word that we added to the dictionary, our grand parents only had a vague idea of what they were and where they came from. Little did they guess that their grand children will be eating, breathing and drinking these pollutants.

Today people are very aware of the toxins in their systems and the need to purge them. Ridding the body of toxins through a detox process will add to our longevity and allow us to lead a happier and healthier life. It was the lack of these toxins that permitted our ancestors to live past the age of 100 while we strive to attain the age of 60. We might just be able to live longer if we detoxify our systems regularly to purge the toxins that accumulate in our systems and wreck havoc with our immune system.

If you observe your life closely you will notice that he food you eat and the liquids you drink comprise of chemicals that are intended to preserver the food and drink. These chemicals inadvertently contribute to the toxin levels in the body when we eat or drink them. The seemingly harmless, aerated drinks, coffee and other processed drinks we consume everyday are crammed with harmful chemicals that will increase the toxins in our body over a period of time. These toxins will ultimately hamper the smooth functioning of he vital organs in the body and will finally lead to bad health and diseases. This is he reason the body must be cleansed of toxins that he system cannot purge by itself.

There are many ways the system can be rid of these toxins. It is called detoxing the body for a healthy mind and body. A popular book called 'The Tao of Detox: The Natural Way to Purify Your Body for Health and Longevity was written by Daniel Reid'. The book is rich with content on how to detox the body through a natural process and is very effective. This book is a must read if you plan to go on a detox diet.

A word of caution though before you go on crash detox diet, consult your physician, though a detox plan is important once a year it must be carried out under the watchful eye of a medical practitioner.

Observe your daily life; most of the food stuffs that you're used to eating contain many harmful chemicals. Beverages like soda pop, coffee, alcohol and other milk beverages can cause certain diseases. Cigarette smokers are not exempted from acquiring harmful acids; as well as inhaling exhaust from cars, trucks, and other vehicles. Dousing yourself with hygiene products which contains harmful chemicals; pharmaceutical drugs, and the modern technology all contributes to acid build up in our body.

So you can just imagine living your life every day with all this harmful things around us. No wonder a lot of people get sick. A call to a natural way of healing diseases or illnesses is the cry of many people who are now aware of the sad fact that many others refuse to believe.

Body detox is a good way to rid your body of the harmful chemicals that has been inside your body for some time now. Detox can help your body to reverse all negative effects from unhealthy lifestyle and eating habits.

There is a lot of detox resources that you can make use to guide you in your quest for a rejuvenated and new life. The book entitled The Tao of Detox: The Natural Way to Purify Your Body for Health and Longevity was written by Daniel Reid. This book will show you a holistic approach to cleanse your body. There is a need to detoxify our internal body, just as it is needed to clean our environment (and the whole planet).

This book will provide you with a solution to restore and preserve good health. And this will only be realized through detoxification. If you desire to live a long life, purchase this book, and let it be your guide to detox your body, and help you change your unhealthy lifestyle. Start now before it is too late.

Detox Diets 101: Keeping Your Body In Shape Through Proper Eating

A feeling of sluggishness accompanied by a feeling of having a permanently full belly and sometimes indigestion are all signs that it is time to detoxify your system. Sometimes you might feel that you are overweight and obese and if you find that your liver may be complaining of excessive toxins, you must sit up and take note as this might be a wake up call for you.

A very common feeling is that of feeling like bring up or a slight nauseous feeling when you see very rich food such as fried stuff or very sweet food. This is a sign that your liver may be unhealthy and that your system needs to be cleansed – and fast. This is the time to figure out and go on a detox diet for a while and give your body time to rejuvenate.

Detoxification is a systematic plan of reducing if not completely removing harmful toxins from the system. There are many detox plans that one may resort to if they need to cleanse the system of harmful toxins. The best plans are the natural plans and consist of detox diets that last from 5 to 10 days. There also detox exercise plans along with the diet that assist the body to get back into shape. You may have detox massages, medication and yoga but the best laid plans that cannot go wrong is the detox diet plan.

A detox diet plan is a plan that will teach you how to eat and what to eat apart from when to eat. All these parameters are equally important and need to be learnt. When you know the right food that can help you lead a healthy life you might just stick to eating healthy. This way you will not need to detoxify your system for years.

A detox diet consists of mainly organic food. This food is mainly green leafy vegetables and fruit. Without the harmful ingredients such as preservatives and additives the food is naturally accepted without the body having to go all out to eliminate the harmful chemicals that go into processing meats and processed foods. Natural food is rich in antioxidants, vitamins and minerals these are much needed for the development of a healthy mind and body. Then there are the natural fibers these foods provide the body. These fibers are very necessary for the body to repair tissue.

There is some caution that needs to be observed while on a detox diet though. If you are planning on getting pregnant or already are, it is best that you stick to the diet you are used to until after you have recuperated from your delivery. You will need all the energy you can get. A detox diet will be a drastic change that your body may not be able to take.

So if you are thinking of starting a detox diet do confer with your medical service provider first. Remember that too much of a good thing is bad too. However, there are many advantages of detoxification and it should be tried at least once a year.

All Natural Body Detox For Body Cleansing And Total Mind Rejuvenation

The term 'toxin' will naturally get the reader to think of a bottle of poison that is not meant to be consumed. The problem is that not all toxins are bottled and soled with a warning label on it. Many a time we consume toxins in our food and drinks without even suspecting it for a moment, these are microscopic bacteria and pollutants that are inadvertently mixed with out food as processing agents and preservatives, which build up over the years and cause problems within out biological systems.

There is another way that pollutants of toxins enter our body. They are available all over the place, in the air we breathe and the water we drink. Toxins can penetrate our skin through the pores and through our lungs by he air we breathe. These pollutants must be removed from our system before they begin to cause problems with our health and well being. The body has to be detoxified at regular intervals and we can do this by periodically following a detox diet.

Many people ask, "Why is the body unable to rid itself of the toxins we take in?" The answer is simple. The human body is capable of cleansing the system to a limited extent. In time the levels of pollution has risen to uncontrollable limits and the body is incapable of handling these levels of toxins. This is why we need to eat wisely and detoxify our systems regularly.

In times gone by our parents used to give us purgatives on a regular basis to rid the body of toxins. We were also encouraged to drink a lot of water, which, by the way was pure. This is something we must pass on to our children. The better way to eat healthy food instead of processed stuff that goes around today.

There is no doubt that the safest way to rid the system of toxins is to detoxify it with a natural process. To do this one must stop eating junk food. Junk food is food that is full of preservatives and in most cases contains a lot of oil and grease. Another name for junk food is 'fast food'. Products such as alcohol, fats, caffeine are all food that add to the toxin levels in the body. A diet that consists of fibrous fruit and vegetables purge out toxins from the body in a very natural and safe way without the use of medications.

Body Detox Made Easy!

It is best to keep off meats and high toxin foods and stick with the healthy fruit and vegetable diet to keep the toxins out in the first place. It may be ok to eat meat and consume alcohol a couple of times in the month but keep it to a minimum if you want to live a healthy life.

Body Detox Made Easy!

When To Say That Detox Diet Guide On Cleansing Your Body Is Safe

During the course of the day we are exposed to many toxins in the atmosphere. Add to this the fact that the water we are consuming day in and day out is not the purest of drinks to quench our thirst. Then there are the various preservatives we are eating along with the food we eat. All this adds up as toxins in our system.

Toxins in our system only contribute to ill health and need to be removed. We remove toxins from our system by following a planned detox regime that may last from 5 days 2 weeks. A detox diet is a diet that comprises of food stuff that are natural in all aspects. This means we have to eat food that is not processes at all, or if need be they must be cooked as little as possible.

Such a detox diet can only consist of a diet of fruit and vegetables that are not cooked in oils, fats and have no preservatives added. Sticking to such a diet for a period of 5 days will clean the system of toxins and leave the body rejuvenated and healthier. It is equally important to drink at least three liters of water a day during the detox regime.

It is common to hear of celebrities taking to detox diets and also people who are getting out of their habit of consuming excessive alcohol. Detox diets are the best way to cleanse the system of toxins that seem to accumulate over the years or even months depending on the level of pollution. You would wonder how safe detox diets are. It is a fact that detox diets do have side effects if the diet is not controlled properly. A safe rule of thumb to follow is to just stick to a fruit and boiled vegetable diet with plenty of water for at lease 8 days. Such a diet will cleanse the system of all the harmful toxins and leave the body free and healthy.

The body does have a natural way of ridding the body of toxins. It does this by processing the food and drink we take in daily and eliminates the toxins in the form of urine, excreta and sweat. The kidneys, liver and intestines are mainly responsible for eliminating the body of toxins. This is, however, true to the amount of toxins the body absorbs. When the levels go up the body needs a little help from us in cleansing the system of these harmful pollutants.

Remember to chew your food completely when dieting or even on a regular basis. It is healthy to chew your food well before swallowing. Remember the lesson in school? Chew your food 32 times before swallowing it? It is true. You need to chew your food. You should plan a diet of brown bread, little rice and a lot of fiber. Cut down on the intake of sugar and spices and drink a lot of water and you will find a marked difference in your level of health and well being.

A Rejuvenating 5-Day Body Detox Plan To Keep You Going

In the present times and age it is impossible to get away from the factors that contribute to the toxification of your system. Pollution is the main cause and you can be sure to find pollution in all spheres of your life. Be it at work, a public place and in the food you eat also the water you during aids in the toxifying process to some extent.

In public places it is imperative to bump into a smoker who will care little for the smoke you inhale due to his or her smoking. The perfumes and toilet sprays are another source of toxins that we end up inhaling and adding to the already present toxins in our system. So what do we do to get rid of these toxins? And what are the ill effects of the toxins in the first place?

Toxins in the body are harmful to an extent that cannot be imagined. For starters toxins in the body speed up the aging process such as wrinkling of the skin apart from causing a lot of illnesses and diseases such as skin rashes and upsetting the digestive process. Though the body has it's own natural process of ridding the body of the toxins there are some toxins that need a little help in the eviction process. The body by itself cannot handle an endless amount of toxins in the body and so needs a little help from us.

It is important to undergo a detoxification process every once in a while. This helps us live a healthier life as well as enjoy our relationship with others around us through a healthy mind. When the pollutants overburden the system the tissues are stressed out and the organs begin to malfunction. This is when a detoxification process is needed.

It is not wise to wait for the body to begin demanding a cleansing process before we begin one. We should undergo a body detoxification once every few months. A simple 5 day detox plan will go a long way in helping the body cleanse itself.

During the 5 day detoxification process certain foods need to be avoided. You should try to consume fresh green vegetables and a lot of fruit. It is important to avoid oils, fats and preservatives and also any food with unnatural additives as these substances contribute greatly to the toxification process. The 5 day detox plan rules out the consumption of meat products completely. So go on a vegetable and fruit diet without the oils and you will have detoxified your system in a matter of 5 days. You will begin to feel the difference in health from the 3rd day of the 5 day detox plan, and the feeling is great!

Body Detox Made Easy!

Gentler Ways To Detox The Body

Toxins come into the body through anything we eat drink or breathe. Toxins also enter the body through the pores of the skin from the water we bathe with and the air we live in. These toxins drain us of all our energy and induce body aches telling us that it is time to detox our system.

If you want to have a clearer skin texture, with renewed levels of energy along with a stronger immune system and an overall sharper mind than you have to consider detoxifying your system through the many procedures available to you. This process is mainly a cleansing process of the blood where the toxins are removed. The cleansing system mainly includes the kidneys, liver and the lymphatic system.

How Do You Detox Your Body?
If you are interested in cleansing your system of toxins then you first have to stop consuming alcohol and smoking cigarettes. You will also need to stop consuming fats, refined foods, brews such as coffee and aerated drinks. These are all contributors of toxins and need to be eliminated before the purification process is started.

Then there are the other sources of toxins that need to be controlled. These are cleaners that are used in households and health products; these include chemical shampoos, deodorants and toothpaste. The toxic chemicals in these products end up in our system and wreck havoc. Though there re a number of ways to detox your system you must choose and decide which way suits you best.

1. **Fasting.** This is the most popular way to rid the body of the harmful toxins that cause disease and suffering. When we never knew the meaning of the word 'toxin' our ancestors used to fast on every Friday to cleanse the system.
2. One of the best ways of detoxing the body is to go on a fruit and vegetable juice diet. Vegetables such as carrots, spinach, celery and cabbage along with fruit juice such as juice from apples, pineapple will rid the system of toxins, however you will need to stick to this juice diet for at least 5 days and remember not to during citrus fruit juice.
3. Lose weight through fasting and exercise. Obese people are known to have the highest levels of toxins in their system. If you go on a juice fast for a period of 30 days you can lose at least 30 pounds of excessive weight.

4. Go on a week long vegetarian diet that includes a lot of green leafy vegetables and a lot of fruit. Remember to drink a lot of water, at least 4 liters per day.

With the proper detox regime you will be able to rid your system of all the toxins in your system leaving you a healthier and more productive person.

Balancing Ph-Ion And Detox To Cleanse The Body

Grow, glow, and go! pH levels indicate the amount of acidity-alkalinity in your body. When your body's pH level becomes too acidic, you may become exhausted, gain weight, suffer poor digestion, and have more aches. If pH is to acidic for longer periods of time, you may suffer more serious problems. If this happens, it would be a good idea to "detox," that is, to reduce the amount of unhealthy toxins in your body and return the pH balance to a more natural alkaline state.

While the human body naturally removes toxins through the processing of blood and waste elimination, it can sometimes be overloaded with unhealthy toxins. This may happen when a person is sick, and his or her biological processes are not functioning properly. It can also happen when we don't maintain a healthy diet. Eating too many acidic foods can produce an unhealthy imbalance. Lack of exercise can also impede your body's ability to clean itself of harmful toxins. No matter how it happens, detoxing can produce a better health and a more productive life generally.

Human bodies work as hard to maintain a healthy blood pH level as they do to maintain a normal temperature. Naturally, our bodies work to maintain a blood pH level of a little more than 7. To do this, it will even stress tissues and internal organs to a proper pH balance. So, you can even be unhealthy because of pH level even when your pH level is in normal ranges.

As mentioned, being overly tired, gaining weight, poor digestion, and aches and pains may indicate that your pH balance is out of whack and your body may be trying to process too many acids. You may be eating too much acid, your body may be creating too much acid, or your body may not be eliminating acids as it should.

One of the easiest ways to detox these acids is to change your diet. Foods that contribute to acidity include dairy products, processed sugars, red meat, alcohol, coffee, and carbonated beverages. If you eat a lot of these, you may be overloading your body beyond its natural ability to neutralize the acids and return to a more normal alkaline state.

Acidifying toxins can also be formed by microforms (microscopic animal or vegetable organisms) and pathogens inside the body. All human bodies contain microscopic organisms that aid digestion, but too many of these microforms may create more acids than the body can handle, impeding digestion and eventually leading to serious conditions like irritable bowel syndrome, Chrohn's disease, and perhaps even colon cancer. These pathogens can enter the blood stream and carry disease with them through the blood to cells, tissues, and entire biologic systems. An out-of-balance pH level may indicate that this is occurring.

These toxins can be removed through a process of detoxification, but an overloaded system can't do it naturally. You'll have to help to return to a healthy pH balance. A detox diet includes highly-alkaline foods like vegetables and low-sugar fruits, focused hydration through drinking lots of water (preferably alkaline water), and proper alkaline-rich supplements.

You can purchase alkalizing products that will help return your normal pH balance. Tasteless, odorless structured alkaline waters are designed for maximum absorption and contain minerals to help achieve a healthy pH balance. They help neutralize acids and remove toxins. When you're using alkaline waters as a first step in a detox diet, you should drink from three to four liters (about 3-4 quarts) every day.

Dietary alkaline supplements contain essential minerals like calcium, magnesium, and iron that replenish your body's mineral reserves and buffer the acids. Some of these mineral-rich supplements will also encourage proper elimination of acids from the body. Though these supplements are relatively new to the market, you can find them at these companies: Innerlight, Phion Nutrition, Vaxa, and Alkalife. But before you begin a detox diet or take supplements, visit your doctor to be sure your problems are correctly diagnosed and the treatments are appropriate.

Body Detox Made Easy!

Cleanse Yourself And Do Body Detox For Better Health

If you're hearing more about body detox these days, it's no accident. Detox ain't just for drugs or alcohol. It's for all of us. We live in a world of air pollution, water pollution, and bad habits. The chemical revolution is still going on, and chemicals, both healthy and not, surround us everywhere.

The US Department of Health and Human Services, through the Centers for Disease Control, performs a survey called NHanes that assesses the health and nutritional status of adults and children in the United States through interviews and direct physical examinations. They found that, in 2003-2004, two-thirds of adults in the U.S. were overweight or obese. Almost 20% of teenagers were found to be overweight or obese.

In today's busy life, we bombard our bodies with fast food, processed food, and a mountain of preservatives and additives every day. And now, we hear about genetically altered "designer" foods whose impact on our bodies is still largely unknown.
Despite the popular focus on health and lifestyle choices, most of us are walking a very thin line when it comes to our diet. The current obesity epidemic is clear evidence that our diets and our lifestyle are out of control. Given this bleak picture, the good news is that people are becoming more aware of the foods they eat.

When we talk about "detoxification," we're talking about the process of removing toxins from our bodies. For our purposes in this article, body detox refers to the use of diets, herbs, and other processes to remove toxins and achieve better health.

If you're concerned about your health and the amount of toxins you may be carrying around with you, it may be time to consider body detox. It's a healthy choice in an otherwise unhealthy world. But don't be fooled. Body detox means a change in lifestyle. It means eating a more balanced combination of healthy, natural foods. It means drinking more water and less coffee and soda. It means regular exercise. It means avoiding fast food, junk food, and processed prepared meals (including frozen dinners and canned goods). These changes will not be easy, and you probably won't want to take it all on at once. But you can begin today to change the way you approach food.

Body Detox Made Easy!

Changing your lifestyle and undertaking body detox also means more and more regular exercise. You don't have to join a gym and buy a bunch of new exercise clothes. You just need to get up and move more! Take brisk walks, go bowling, walk when you want to ride, carry your own groceries to the car. There are a million ways to get more exercise without even noticing it.

If you're more serious about detoxing your body, you may want to investigate a detox diet. It will reduce the toxins in your body, relieve aches and pains, reduce the discomfort of allergies, improve digestive problems, and increase your energy level. You can find many body detox recipes on the internet. A trip to your local health food store is also a good way to learn about body detox foods and recipes.

When you're committed to body detox, eat as many fresh fruits as you can. Favor nuts, beans, rice, and grains over fried foods and gravy. And try to avoid sugary desserts, caffeine, alcohol, yeast-rich dishes, and processed foods that contain many questionable preservatives and additives.

A one- or two-day fast is a good way to transition in and out of your body detox effort. Be sure to get plenty of liquids, especially water, during your fast. And don't push it. If hunger becomes an obsession, have a piece of fruit or a few carrots or celery sticks. You don't have to punish yourself during your body detox.

There are many other ways to detox and to change your lifestyle to one that promotes personal health and happiness. Re-acquaint yourself with nature. Go outdoors and enjoy the fresh air. Take a long walk at the beach or in your neighborhood park or nature preserve. Incorporate "me time" into your daily schedule, and make it a family affair too. Keep active and interested in the world around you. Get involved.

For a real body detox treat, go to the spa. Have a relaxing massage or deep-cleaning facial. When you shower, use a brush to accelerate the detox process. Brushing your skin gently will improve your circulation and help you shed those layers of toxin-rich dead skin.

Help your body eliminate toxins naturally. Drink at least four quarters (or liters) of water every day. Eat fiber-rich foods like raspberries, blackberries, broccoli, apples (with the skin), spinach,

Body Detox Made Easy!

almonds or peanuts, and good old stone-ground whole wheat. And when you stop by that health food store, look for teas and other herbs that will encourage regular bowel movements.

Body detox involves some mind detox too. Negative thinking, believe it or not, contributes to the production of toxins and over-acidity in the body. Rid yourself of worry, anger, and pessimism. They serve no positive purpose, and they are unhealthy. Smile until you want to smile.

There's no bad time to start body detox. Today's hurried, high-stress pace cries out for a little personal self-care. And your family deserves the same healthy lifestyle. Body detox may be as simple as working on your attitude, ridding yourself of negative, destructive thinking that compromises your health. It can be as easy as taking a walk in the park or treating yourself to a long, hot shower. It can also be as complex as adopting and sticking to a strict detox diet that cleans your tissues and organs of harmful pathogens and over-acid chemistry. It's your choice. The important thing is finding a way to cleanse yourself.

Whatever approach you choose, you're doing yourself and those around you a favor. You're bringing some sanity back into your life and setting an example for your children and your social circle. You're living better and enjoying life more.

How much would you pay to have that miracle? Well, you don't have to pay a thing! You just have to change your approach to your day - each and every day.

Body Detox: The Process To Purify Your Life, Mind, And Soul

Human bodies must be detoxified. That is, the amount of toxins and pathogens must be removed from the body in order to maintain health and happiness. A healthy human body removes toxins through normal biological processes and waste elimination. But in today's environment, our bodies are bombarded with pollutants that compromise health and the immune system. Body detox is a process through which we intentionally change, at the very least, our food and lifestyle choices to allow the body to process and reduce toxins and pathogens to a safe level.

The primary cause of toxin build-up is poor diet. Fast food, junk food, and the preservatives and additives in processed foods lead to any number of complaints as they throw bodily processes out of whack. Among the most harmful foods are those high in acidity like caffeine, carbonated beverages, meat, sugary foods, and processed (including canned and frozen) foods. Toxin overload can also result when your biological processes are not operating properly, including when you can't eliminate wastes properly. Changing your diet in a good body detox program may allow your biological processes to recover to a normal state.

When toxins within the body exceed normal healthy ranges, a person can become exhausted easily, gain weight, develop muscle and joint pain, and even, in the extreme, develop cancer. Some scientists suggest that the formation of too many free radicals begins a chain reaction that overwhelms the healthy body. We know that an overly acidic pH level in the human body can create these symptoms.

Health is not just physical fitness and being free of disease. The chemicals, hormones, and enzymes in our bodies also affect the way we think and feel emotionally. Recall your mood the last time you were sick. When the body is not healthy, we tend to think more negative thoughts and feel more destructive emotions. As our bodies become more stressed, so do your spirits. And the opposite is true as well. Negative thinking and destructive emotions can attack our health and weaken our resistance to disease. Body detox helps bring purify not only our blood and organs, but our mind and spirit, creating not only better health, but a better life generally.

Short for "detoxification," detox occurs on several levels. Physically, it involves cleaning harmful substances from the system and returning the body to a natural balance. Believe it or not, a health pH balance is as important to our health as maintaining a healthy temperature. There are a variety of body detox diets and programs available that will show you how to promote better health. Search for "detox diet" or "body detox" on the Internet to find an array of options for self-cleansing. Visit your local health food store for more ideas and advice.

Detoxification of the mind is also an important part of a body detox program. Reducing the stress, worry, frustration, and anger in your daily life can speed body detox up and help maintain healthy processes and chemical balances within the body. By attending to your psychological and emotional needs, you can transform stress to joy and transform illness to good health.

Eastern philosophers and religious leaders have long been aware of the importance of physical well-being to spiritual well-being. Fasting, which is an important part of body detox, is an ancient practice that coincidentally helps remove harmful toxins from the body. Doing this makes a person's mind more clear and heart more stable. Though they wouldn't have used the phrase, body detox is a basic part of a healthy spiritual life as well.

Concepts surrounding the process of body detox are relatively new on the science scene. However, many leaders in helping professions for physical, mental, and emotional healing believe that detoxification is essential in today's world. A body detox program including a better diet, more regular physical exercise, and attention to one's mental and emotional states may be one of the most positive changes we can make in our lives today.

Pollution, stress, conflict, and confusion are the hallmarks of modern society. As individuals, we can't do a lot to eliminate larger environmental and social problems. But we can make a big difference one at a time as each of us works to make healthy, positive changes in our lifestyle and in the way we view life. Body detox can do much more than relieve aches and pains or help you lose weight. It can change your life and your outlook on life.

You don't have to undertake a complex, formal body detox program to improve your health. Broad life style changes that may go a long way to restoring your health and outlook include:

- Drinking 3-4 quarters of water every day

Body Detox Made Easy!

- Eating more vegetables and fruit and less meat and dairy

- Increasing the amount of regular physical exercise you get

- Try short fasts (1-2 days)

- Avoid caffeine, sugary desserts, carbonated beverages, alcohol, milk chocolate, and high-acid foods

- Check into available alkalizing water and food supplements to help restore healthy pH balance

- Schedule "me time" every day to restore your mental and emotional balance

- Consider meditation or yoga

A final word of advice. If you've decided to undertake a detox diet or make major changes in your diet or lifestyle, visit your doctor first. Be sure there isn't another physical problem that requires medical treatment before you commit to a formal detox program. Having said that, consider body detox to improve the quality of your and your family's lives.

Healthy Eating With Detox Recipes For Your Body

Many people believe that our bodies are overcome by the toxins in modern civilization. Air and water pollution, chemicals in everyday products, food additives, and cigarette smoke are all sources of toxins that may remain in our bodies when they are not eliminated by our normal biological processes. As a result, we may suffer effects like premature aging, bloating, or obesity.

Detoxification, or detox, is the process of removing toxic substances from the body. A detox diet is the easiest and healthiest way to detox your body. The major DO: more fiber and water are good. The major DON'T: caffeine, carbonated beverages, and sugars (alcohol, chocolate, and yeast) are not good.

One of the most aggressive detox diets, recommended by Dr. Kiki Sidhwa, involves fasting for three days followed by eating only one type of fruit for each meal. For example, breakfast might be an apple. Lunch might consist of oranges or pineapples. Then supper might be either apples or grapes or bananas. You can eat as much of the fruit as you want during each meal. Snacks might be a type of fruit non-sweetened fruit juice. The most important point is not to mix your fruit. Eat only one type of fruit for each meal.

If this approach is too extreme, you might want to use some detox diet recipes. They're designed to give you the nutrients you need and the antioxidants that will clean your body of toxins. Increasing your intake of fluids is a great way to begin your detox diet.

Ginger Healing Tea with Tumeric is a delicious and effective addition to a detox diet. Ginger contains many antioxidants that may prevent cancer. It is known to cure nausea, motion sickness, and morning sickness. Boil two cups of water and add: 1/2 tsp. of powdered ginger, 1/2 tsp. of turmeric. Let the mixture simmer for ten minutes, then strain the tea into a mug, adding one tablespoon of maple syrup and a dash of lemon extract.

Vegetable super-juice makes a great detox diet breakfast. It gives you an energy boost, wakes up your digestive system, and keeps you powered through lunch. Ingredients include a whole cucumber, four sticks of celery, about an ounce of fresh spinach, and eight leaves of lettuce. Other green vegetables (parsley or fresh alfalfa sprouts) make a healthy addition to the super-juice. Use a blender or beverage maker to puree the ingredients, adding an equal amount of distilled water to aid the process. Lemon juice will add a tart and interesting taste. Even though cucumbers are less nutritious than most fruit, cucumber seeds are a good source of vitamins A, B6, C and K. Cucumbers also contain potassium, thiamin, folate, pantothenic acid, magnesium, phosphorus, copper, and manganese.

For lunch, try a high-energizing detox diet soup that is a favorite for detox diets. Combine one avocado with two spring onions, a half red or green pepper, a cucumber, a half-ounce of fresh spinach, half a clove of garlic and about one-third cup of yeast-free vegetable bouillon. Add the juice of one lemon or lime and, if you want, add a little coriander, cumin, or parsley. Blend the avocado and vegetable bouillon until it forms a paste, and then add the other ingredients. Soup's on!

A wonderful detox diet dinner treat is Warm Broccoli Soup. Start by lightly steaming (5-6 minutes) six to eight good-sized broccoli heads. Put the steamed broccoli into a blender with one-half an avocado, one-third of a red onion, one stick of celery, a handful of raw spinach, an inch of ginger root. Blend well and then add cumin, Bragg liquid amino, garlic, and ground black pepper for taste. This cold weather favorite is an excellent way to return your body's chemical balance to its naturally alkaline state.

These are just a few of the many detox diet recipes you can find on the Internet. The most important part of this process is getting lots of water and essential nutrients while also avoiding harmful food additives and preservatives and the sugar most modern processed foods are loaded with. Don't put it off another day! Eat healthy! Start your new healthy life with an effective detox diet.

Home Body-Detox Programs For Losing Weight

There's a lot of attention to weight and having a great body these days. Most of us, no matter what we weigh, probably think we could stand to lose a few pounds. The U.S. Centers for Disease Control has found that two-thirds of adults, and almost one-fifth of teens, are overweight or obese. If you've ever tried to diet, you know how frustrating it can be in adding or getting rid of a few pounds. In truth, most diets don't work because they don't get to the root of the problem - poor habits and compromised health.

Since the day we were born, our bodies have been accumulating toxins. And in today's world, we are bombarded with them. Not only are we overwhelmed by fast food and processed meals, our environment is burdened by air and water pollution and a range of modern chemicals. And more recently, genetic engineering of foods has made keeping healthy an even greater mystery.

But the number one offender is diet. Our bodies are designed to eliminate toxins and maintain health balances of temperature, pH level, and biological processes. There are three main ways we eliminate toxins naturally: through a more alkaline (than acidic) diet, through biologic processes that restore health balance internally, and through elimination of wastes through the digestive process. When our diets are overly acidic, the normal processes are over-stressed, and we begin to suffer symptoms like exhaustion, muscle and tissue pain, weight gain, and eventually more serious diseases (even cancer).

If you're experiencing these symptoms, or if you are generally feeling less that healthy, you may need to detoxify your body. Many scientists and health-care workers think home body detox is a practical, rational solution for restoring healthy chemical balances within the body.

A successful detox program can help you lose weight, restore your energy, reduce symptoms of asthma and diabetes, and slow down the aging process. Home body detox is an attractive alternative to popular diets because it focuses first on you health and, second, on your weight. Improving your health is the best way to achieve long-term weight loss, and it may be less expensive that the diets you see advertised in the market today. And while you're losing weight, the home body detox program is enhancing your body's natural ability to cleanse itself, bringing it back to a healthy balance.

Body Detox Made Easy!

It's easy to practice your body detox program at home, since most of its aspects involve food choices and personal habits. You can detoxify your body without special prescriptions or medications, though you may want to add some alkalizing water or vitamin/mineral supplements to speed the detox process. Effective home body detox programs can be accomplished in as little as two to three weeks.

The goals of a home body detox program is to help you lose weight, improve circulation, increase toxin elimination, cleanse the colon, and provide nutrients to the liver. Your liver is the primary organ for natural detoxification, and liver health should be one of your top priorities.

People who've followed home body detox programs report they there were able to lose weight faster than they had with other diets and weight-loss products. They also reported clearer skin, better digestion, more energy, and more regular bowel movements.

By practicing home body detox, you'll learn what foods support your health. Fresh fruit and vegetables are highly recommended for both weight loss and bringing your pH level to a more normal, healthy alkaline state. Fresh low-sugar fruit, leafy green vegetables, alkalized water, virgin oils, stone-ground whole wheat products, lemon water, and non-caffeinated, non-carbonated drinks should replace the old processed meals, canned goods, meat- and dairy-heavy meals, and alcohol. And be sure to drink more water. During a home body detox program, experts recommend at least 4 quarts of water each day. After detox, you should still be sure to drink at least two quarts a day. Short one- and two-day fasts will also speed up the body detox process.

Another reason to undertake a home body detox program is that you will learn new, healthy habits that will extend well belong your weight-loss period. It's important to know that, if you return to your old eating habits, your body will begin to retain toxins, and you'll eventually find yourself with unwanted symptoms, including weight gain. Maintaining a proper diet will help your body process and eliminate toxins naturally and effectively without supplements or medications. It's your choice. Live healthy and have a healthy life. Live unhealthy and make unhealthy lifestyle choices, and you'll be back to the home body detox program.

You don't have to embark on all these changes at once. You can start slowly by changing some eating habits now and others later. Begin getting more and more regular exercise by taking short walks, leading up eventually to a more aggressive exercise program. Detox your mind, too. Schedule private time each day to maintain a healthy psychological and emotional balance to reduce the stresses that add to ill health.

One last word of advice: before you start any diet or home body detox program, visit your doctor to be sure you don't have a more serious problem that should be treated medically before undertaking home body detox. Your doctor may be able to give you additional advice that will enhance body detox and help lead you to a new healthy, happy lifestyle.

Body Detox Made Easy!

Detox Body In 7 Days With Internal Cleansers

Being aware of diseases and illnesses and what causes them is a great way of staying away from them. Today, medical costs are increasing and getting sick is an expensive business. This is one reason why people want to remain healthy. But are people ready to make some compromises to achieve this? Staying healthy involves eating the correct food in the correct amount and at the correct time, and avoiding harmful habits like alcohol and cigarettes. Health needs you to change your lifestyle as much as possible. If you think you are up to it, then rest assured; you can live an illness free and healthy life.

Because of the beverages and food items that you have been eating over the years, your body is susceptible to a number of diseases and illnesses. Even the environment around you can affect the toxin level in your body. Toxin build up happens when the toxic content goes over what the body's natural detoxification process can handle. This kind of toxic build up causes a lot of problems for the body and this leads to sickness.

The detox diet consisting of natural herbs and supplements is gaining a lot of popularity these days. These foods help the body get rid of toxins through the liver, lungs, skin, kidneys and the intestines. Toxins are also eliminated by the body's lymphatic system.

However, you must consult your doctor before you prescribe any detox diet program because only a doctor can assess your present health situation and tell you if what you are planning is safe.

If you are already experiencing a toxic build up, there are definite symptoms that can point to it. And on starting your detox regime, these symptoms tend to get worse. But you must keep patience because this condition will pass in a few days. In fact it is a good sign as it signifies that your body is undergoing detoxification.

If you are searching for a neat way of getting rid of the toxins present in your body, you can try the detox body cleanser. It has been proven to clean up your body's internal parts in just 7 days.

You can start a seven-day detox program for yourself using the body cleanser and eliminate all the unwanted toxins present in your body. The detox body cleanser can either come as a fiber

Body Detox Made Easy!

packet or in the tablet form. It contains natural herbs and fibers. In seven days you will feel visibly energized, revitalized and detoxified. There are people who have even claimed to see effects after just the first day.

These detox body cleansers are usually reasonably priced, usually around $12. but if a healthy body is what you wish to achieve, price should not be such a heavy consideration.

Detox body cleansers are simple to use and even though they are made of various herbs, they are great to taste and so it is easy to digest too. These cleansers aim at giving your entire body a good cleansing and this is what it does.

Detox body cleansers can be found at all leading drugstores. You can even buy it at an online store. Try the seven-day body cleanser to get fast results.

Body Detox Made Easy!

Body Detox- The Elemis Silhouette Body Contouring Capsule

In today's world and with the lifestyle that people lead, it is very easy for toxins to find a way into our bodies and settle there until we make an effort to remove them. Before you know it, your body has been polluted and has started to deteriorate and you are only left with the symptoms. But the good part is, it is never too late to make an effort to make your body healthy again.

If you are experiencing a sluggishness or weakness of the body along with frequent headaches, indigestion, coughing etc, then your body is probably infested with toxins. Although sometimes, they might be symptoms of some disease, very often they can be traced to the presence of some toxin in the body. If you don't get rid of the toxins, they can cause a lot of problems.

Take, for instance, indigestion and slow metabolism. They cause food not being digested properly and this leads to stagnant fat. This causes weight gain in people, which in some severe case leads to obesity. Added to this is the feeling of sluggishness that causes you to eat more even when you are not hungry. Often people are misled by the notion that eating a lot of food can provide the body with energy. It is not insufficient intake of food that weakens the body; it's the toxins.

If in such cases, you detoxify your body, your body develops and you sweat away the excess fat. The Elemis Silhouette body contouring detox capsule works in this principal. These capsules help in promoting good digestion and in enhancing the metabolism to flush the toxins away. These capsules also rejuvenate and maintain the body so that it gives you the confidence you require to meet daily challenges.

The Elemis Silhouette contouring capsules contain Centella Asiatica, Laminaria algae and Klamath Lake algae that are known to provide the body with protein supplements, purify the blood and enhance digestion of fat. These detox capsules contain cellulite programs that use advance science proven to be efficient and safe. The formulas used in the capsules have undergone a number of tests and examinations, which is why it is recommended by a lot of nutritionists.

The best part of the capsule is that there is no requirement for you to starve or fast to achieve the desired results. You eat a sufficient meal along with two capsules during breakfast. Once the effect has been achieved, you can cut it down to only one tablet. In order to facilitate the process of detoxification, you should drink loads of water along with the capsule. Just like any other capsule, certain precautionary methods should be taken while taking this treatment. Prior to taking any medicine, consult your doctor, especially if you are pregnant, are a lactating mother, a diabetic, or suffer from high blood pressure. Reduce the dosage in case you experience nausea or any other allergy repeatedly.

People of any skin type, be it dry or oily, can take the Elemis Silhouette Body detox capsule. But children below 18 are advised not to take this capsule. The Elemis Silhouette detox capsule can rejuvenate, detox and reshape you, all in a healthy and hassle free manner that suits your lif est yle.

Body Detox The Easy Way: A Natural Diet

You may wonder sometimes why your body seems to be heavy and you feel lazy to move, yet you are not sick. You are more than willing to be energetic but your body is not just up to it. To address the problem, you resort to eating a lot, gulp up cups of coffee and smoke, thinking that you will be lively after. For a while, you feel good and going. Unknowingly though, you are accumulating toxins in your body. With this scenario happening more and more, you might need to detoxify.

With our ever-dynamic world today, we want our bodies to be constantly active so we can move along with the fast paced lifestyles. Hence, we resort to body stimulants such as coffee, cigarettes, diet pills, drugs and a lot more thinking that they will help the body to stay up all the time, but they do otherwise. These stimulants cause immediate loss of energy and emotional symptoms such as headaches, sickness and depression. They are also considered as toxins in the body.

What are toxins? Toxins are agents that are able to cause body harm. There are two kinds of toxins, the Exogenous or external toxins and Endogenous or internal toxins. The Exogenous toxins come from external sources such as car fumes, tobacco smoke, drugs, factory pollution, etc. On the other hand, the Enogenous toxins come from viral or bacterial infection. Due to metabolism, the body creates its own toxin called Autogenous toxins.

These harmful substances are eliminated in the body in a process called detoxification. Detoxification is the removal of stored toxic products from the bowel, the blood, liver, and kidneys including the great amount of toxic substances stored in body fat to cure chronic diseases such as cancer. The easiest way to detoxify the body is the body detox through a natural diet. To detoxify the body naturally is a change in the diet from a poor to a healthy one. A healthy diet includes raw food diet, specifically, fruits and vegetables.

Naturally, the body detoxifies itself all day. The peak of detoxification occurs when the body is rested during sleep until noon. This is a way for the body to eliminate the toxins acquired from pollution, stimulants and nutrients.

Body Detox Made Easy!

For the ever busy people, you can substitute your stimulants with natural diet to acquire a healthy and active body. Most common stimulants taken by people are refined white sugar, coffee, diet pills, cigarettes and red meat.

Sugar has a stimulating effect. Hence, we feel invigorated when we drink colas. What we do not know, refined white sugar has detrimental effects on the body. Examples of products containing refined white sugar are cola and ketchup. It is advised to cut down on it by using brown sugars like cane sugar which is natural. Fruit juices also give the same kick as to refined white sugar. Late night workers resort to drinking coffee to keep them awake. As natural substitute to coffee with a detoxifying effect is Japanese or Chinese green tea. The Japanese or Chinese green tea gives the same kick because it also contains caffeine but it does not contain substances that are irritating to the stomach.

Diet pills are also stimulants for the body to be kept alive. This may be observed among athletes specially, during time for competitions because they give more energy. They are being taken albeit the toxic effect in the body. In lieu of this, athletes must take fruits instead due to their natural detoxifying effects.

For cigarette smokers who think smoking stimulates their mind to think, they must think twice for smoking causes cancer. If they take carrots, they will experience the same effect in a more natural way.

For red meat lovers who really feel good and strong after feasting on said food, they better think about cutting on it. Fish is a better substitute.

Now, we understand why our parents keep on reminding us to eat fruits and vegetables. They give us energy in more natural ways plus they keep us fit and healthy.

Detox- The Natural Way

There maybe times when your body feels too heavy and you feel too lethargic to move even though there is nothing physically wrong with you. You want to do something energetic but your body is slack and you can't bring yourself to engage in activity. As a solution to this, you resort to lots of food and smoke and think this might make you feel lively again. All these habits have only temporary effect and the only thing you are doing is increasing toxin accumulation in your body.

With today's changing world, we too want our bodies to be ever dynamic and ready for activity as and when required. Therefore we settle for body stimulants like cigarettes, coffee, drugs, diet pills and other things thinking that all these things will keep our body active all the time but this is not true. These kinds of stimulants cause loss of energy and lead to emotional symptoms like sickness, depression and headaches. They also leave toxins in the body.

Toxins are substances that cause harm to the body. Generally, there are two types of toxins- the internal or endogenous toxins and the external or exogenous toxins. External toxins arise out of external sources like tobacco smoke, car fumes, factory pollution, drugs etc. Similarly, bacterial or viral infections are sources of internal toxins. The body manufactures its own set of toxins known as autogenous toxins.

The body eliminates these harmful substances through a process known as detoxification. Detoxification is responsible for the removal of accumulated toxic products present in the blood, liver, kidneys and bowels as well as the toxic substances present in body fat. The simplest way of getting rid of toxins is through a body detox regime that involves a natural diet, especially vegetables and fruits.

If you usually lead a very busy life then it is time you substitute your stimulants with something more natural to regain energy and strength. The most commonly used stimulants are cigarettes, red meat, diet pills, coffee and refined sugar.

Sugar is known for its stimulating effect. This is the reason colas invigorate us. But we forget that refined white sugar is extremely dangerous for the body. Cola and ketchup contain the maximum amount of refined white sugar. You can cut down on your refined white sugar intake be substituting it with brown sugars and cane sugars which are natural. You can get the same kick out of fruit juices but without the detrimental effect.

People who work late at night often drink coffee in order to stay awake. Instead of coffee, Chinese or Japanese green tea can be drunk, which is much healthier. The Chinese or Japanese green tea contains caffeine and so gives the same kick as coffee, but it does not irritate the stomach.

Often people stimulate themselves by having diet pills in exchange of food. This is a common practice among athletes; especially during competitions as diet pills are known to give energy. They continue consuming these pills even after knowing of their bad effects. These athletes should, instead, eat lots of fruits, as they are good detoxifying agents.

Cigarette smokers often think that cigarette aids the mind in thinking, but all that cigarettes do is cause cancer. Carrot can give the same high as cigarettes but in a much healthier and beneficial manner.

This is why we are encouraged to eat vegetables and fruits from our childhood. It is because they are known to make the body healthy and help it fight and eliminate toxins.

Detox- Why It Is Necessary

In today's world, toxicity has become a matter of great concern. This is due to the fact that today's lifestyle is causing a lot of toxins to accumulate in the human body. The main factors causing this accumulation are air and water pollution, stronger chemicals, radiation and nuclear power. Added to this are all the new chemicals and drugs that people are ingesting along with sugar, refined foods, stimulants and sedatives.

Toxins are a serious problem and can even lead to diseases. Cancer and other cardiovascular illnesses are commonly caused due to increased toxin content in the body. Other illnesses are allergies, obesity, skin problems, arthritis and other health related problems. Also toxin accumulation leads to constant headaches, fatigue, gastrointestinal problems, body pains, coughs as well as other problems that weaken the immune system.

Detoxification or cleansing of the body can help in alleviating these acute and chronic illnesses. The process involves getting rid of the harmful chemicals and toxins present in the body. A detox procedure can either be a short one or a long one. The program especially helps those who are victims of addiction. They are initially kept off their addictive agent and later on they automatically lose their bad habits.

Toxicity has two levels of action. It can either be external or internal. External toxicity is caused due to environmental exposure by breathing, physical contact of ingestion. External also includes the chemicals in foods that we consume. Most drugs, allergens and food additives create toxic elements in the body. There is a certain amount of toxicity present even in nutrients, sodium and water. In contrast, toxins produced internally by the body are internal toxins and occur due to daily normal functions.

Bodily, biochemical and cellular activities produce some substances that need to be eliminated. These free radicals, also called biochemical toxins, cause problems like irritation or inflammation of cells and tissues, which can cause problems in the normal functioning of body cells or organs. A number of foreign bacteria, parasites, intestinal bacteria, yeasts and microbes produce unwanted products that are metabolic. Thoughts, stress and emotions also cause the creation of biochemical toxins.

Body Detox Made Easy!

Just about everybody has to detoxify the body in order for it to function well. Cleansing or detox is the third part of nutritional action. Lesser intensive detoxification is required if you eat a balanced diet and avoid excesses.

Even though the body runs an elimination cycle every morning and night, a diet consisting of refined foods, higher fats, dairy products and drug intake produces a lot of toxin in the body. Because some people lead such lifestyles, body detoxification is important.

Fasting is another detox therapy that people follow. It is one of the most complete and oldest natural human treatments. In a detox process, dead cells and wastes are cleared, the body is revitalized of its natural functions, and the healing capacity of the body is regained. And a lot of people stand proof to the fact that a cleansing program works wonderful results for them.

It is important to a person's health to eliminate toxins in a proper way. Even though the body is capable of handling a certain amount of toxic content, it is best to keep the content low and think of ways of reducing it through our food intake. Detox really works and at the end of it you will find yourself with a better immune system and a healthier body that works well. You will avoid a lot of diseases and hence live a better life.

Detox Foot Patch

With the kind of lifestyle that people live these days, there are numerous avenues through with pollutants and toxins can enter the body. Regularly washing out these toxins and pollutants is a great way of cleaning up the body. One way of body detoxification is using a detox foot patch that works wonders for cleaning the body, both from inside and out.

Remember, a number of environmental factors are responsible for the waste products that have accumulated in the body. These waste products include toxins present in the food we eat and the air we inhale. One excellent way of removing these toxins is by using the detox foot patch.

Basically, a detox foot patch consists of an adhesive patch that is square shaped and is attached under the foot and kept in that position overnight. The reason a detox foot patch is used is for detoxification of the waste products and providing them an outlet that is on the individual's body for a period of time.

Various natural ingredients present in the foot patch are responsible for pulling out the various toxins that cause fatigue, stress and other health problems. People in different regions of Asia use this kind of foot patch. It has spread from Asia to other continents because of the remarkable results shown by the foot patch. All this shows what a great success the foot patch is, not only in Asia but also around the world.

There are a number of advantages of using a foot patch.

· It is an effective method of body detoxification as it treats symptoms of various ailments at a time. It has been proved that people using these patches have shown signs of being more relaxed, restful and many of their minor health problems have been eliminated because of the removal of large amounts of toxin from the body.

· It is comfortable to use. It also gives a person relief from pain. Its main advantage is that it cleans the body. Restfulness, lesser stress and great overall health can be achieved by the complete cleansing of the body.

Body Detox Made Easy!

- It is extremely convenient to use. It can be used at anytime and anywhere. People can use it when they are working or sleeping. It does not hinder any other activity.

- The detox foot patch cleanses the entire body and detoxifies it in a non messy manner.
There are no liquids and ointments involved. All you have to do it stick it under your foot. It is a new and advanced detox gadget and is not known to involve any invasive procedure for body cleansing. This is another reason why it is so popular all over the world and so many people find it suitable.

- It is not at all expensive. It is usually available at a reasonable rate. Usually this treatment can be bought at around 30-40 dollars per box.

Therefore, one can conclude that using the detox foot patch for detoxifying the body is a great way or cleansing the body. There are too many advantages to pass the opportunity to use it. Its results are known to be outstanding and it is best you try it out at least once to avail the benefits of its magic.

How Detox Wrap Works Miracles To Your Body

Looking beautiful from the outside is not the only thing that is essential for feeling good. Almost everybody believes that beauty is only skin deep. Being pretty or beautiful is no guarantee that the person is actually good at heart.

Today, it has become natural for everybody to eat all kinds of food, smoke cigarettes, drink alcohol, and take oral contraceptives and much more. You might not be fully aware of the bad effects of this kind of lifestyle, or perhaps you know but choose to ignore. Toxins enter the body in large amounts on drinking alcohol, eating food items with additives and preservatives etc. toxins are basically chemicals and the body has its own way of getting rid of this in the form of urine and stool. But if these toxins accumulate in the body, in the long run the body will not be able to get rid of these toxins on its own and this can be very harmful for the body. In such cases one has to help the body in the detoxification process. If the condition is let to persist, it can lead to problems like hormonal imbalances, insufficient metabolism, nutritional deficiencies etc. If you are experiencing symptoms like lethargy, occasional pains, dull skin and allergies, you require to detox as soon as possible because these are signs that a lot of toxin has already accumulated inside your body.

For people who want to detox, body wraps are being offered. Body wraps are formulated specially in order to remove toxins from the body. Body wraps are mostly made of sea clay that is known to act as a poultice. The clay helps in drawing out toxins and compressing the tissues of the skin to help regain skins elasticity. Your muscle base becomes smoother and firmer.

How does a body wrap function? Your body has been accumulating toxins for years and years now and they would have built up in and around the fat cells. Depending on your lifestyle, these toxins keep increasing and gaining. The detox body wrap functions by shaping your body by repositioning the fat cells in the body, which also helps in weight loss. If you wish to lose some weight in your buttocks, thighs or any other part of your body, a body wrap can give you almost instant results.

The body wrap moves into the skin pores till it reaches the toxins. These toxins are either flushed out or come back through the wrap. You must ensure that the sea clay you are using is concentrated and if all goes well, in a few days you will be able to notice the inches that you have lost from your body. You might think that the body wrap can cause dehydration of the body but this is not so. You can drink a lot of water without the fear of gaining the lost weight. And you needn't wash off the solution of the wrap. Once you are successful in getting rid of the toxins, there is no way they can return into the body. But if you continue your lifestyle, there is no stopping them from building up inside your body again.

There are a number of detox body wraps available and you can choose any. There are a number of brands for these body wraps too. A lot of these brands promise inch loss in 30 days while others give a full money back guarantee on their product. Anybody can use a detox body wrap. But emphysema phlebitis patients and pregnant women are best advised not to use the wrap.

Detox- For The Mind, Body And Spirit

Today, spirituality has become a vital part of most people's lives. If you are a believer, then you will know the things that you should and shouldn't do. These days, holistic living is becoming extremely popular. This type of lifestyle advocates a healthier and more spiritual life.

People who are highly pious and religious will say that there is no point in having any health if one cannot attain a spiritual high. The body and the mind need to be in sync in order to cleanse the system.

A lot of people say that one must live ones life to the fullest, so why not go for a full body detox? Detoxification or detox is a process in which the harmful chemicals that accumulate in our body are eliminated. The mind, body and spirit are known to be interdependent as neither will function without the other.

It is a pity that people find very little time to spend with their spiritual self. They are too busy paying bills, meeting deadlines, making money, meeting people and trying to keep healthy to pay attention to their spirit. This is all right as everyone has a right to live their life as they please. But if you want to cleanse your entire system, go for a full detox; mind body and soul.

The body usually has its own methods of detoxifying but sometimes when the toxins get too much, the body is not able to handle it on its own. There are detox products sold world over.

Detox products help in the detoxification process and help in revitalizing and energizing the body. Normal bowel movement and healthier skin are other benefits of a body detox.
One has to detox the mind once in a while. You mind has to be freed of all negative thoughts. In the eastern cultures, psychoneurimmunology has been believed to have been practiced for centuries. It states that the body and mind are linked together.

Patients being treated are made to focus on their mind and to visualize healing energy flowing into the organs of the body that needs healing. If you undergo this treatment successfully, it is said that the rate of the healing process moves faster. The key to uniting the body and mind and achieving positive results is visualization. But in order to do this, you need to seek the guidance of professionals who are experienced in mind detox. There are other kinds of mind detox too that can be made use of. You need to choose the one that is best for you.

Spirituality is another part of a person's life that requires attention. Spirituality is exhibited most popularly through the medium of prayer. Prayer is a part of almost all religions all over the world. There is no correct way of praying and nobody can tell you how to do it. You can pray wherever you like, any way you choose to, just as long as its genuine and is backed by faith. All that is required is finding a method of prayer that you find suitable and after that you are ready for your spiritual detox.

These are ways of getting a full mind, body and spirit detox and these are just some of the ways. You can always seek professional guidance if you want to make sure you get it right.

Detox- Bruce Fife Tells You How

Wealth is absolutely of no good if one cannot keep good health. If the body doesn't function well and keeps falling ill, one cannot enjoy life at all. You might just miss out on some great events and opportunities because of bad health. Without knowing, you are bombarding your body with many harmful chemicals. These harmful chemicals can make your body weak over a period of time and affect your daily activity. It, therefore, becomes important to make efforts to get rid of these harmful chemicals.

You might ask where these chemicals are coming from. In case you haven't guessed, all these harmful chemicals come from the food and drinks you have consumed, and other daily consumptions like fumes and smoke from cigarettes and cars and other sources. Every day you are exposing your body to these harmful chemicals contained in almost everything around you.

Although the body has its own process of self-healing and toxin elimination, in some situations it is incapable of doing it alone especially if the body has already has an acid build up. Acid build up happens due to an unhealthy lifestyle for a prolonged period of time. If you have been living an unhealthy life it is time you give your body a detoxification and you do it fast. If you keep putting it off for later, you will start experiencing symptoms of illnesses and diseases. One suggestion is buying a book by Bruce Fife on body detox. You can get help from the expert himself and start detoxifying your body for just $20.

Consumers have given great ratings for this book in different reviews. This book tells us everything we need to know about detox. It helps you decide on regimens that can facilitate the elimination of toxins and harmful substances from the body. As is commonly known, the air one inhales also contains toxins. So does the food we eat. The body produces some toxins if it is not functioning properly and they cannot be ousted and this causes a lot of problems later on.

This book contains all the information needed for you to decide how to go about the detox program at home. Some support is required for the natural detoxification of the body's system, and home detox programs can help in the eliminating diseases that you might have developed, restoring the body's health and in reversing signs of aging and other problems that people face. This rejuvenates the body and helps you regain your energy once again.

The book also features a diet that contains all natural foods. This book gives you lessons on the good affects of fasting, how to go about it and other ways of detoxifying the body in as natural a way as possible.

However, the book has a few drawbacks. The author is a vegetarian and so some issues related to eating toxin free food have been addressed a little partially and this does not sit well for non-vegetarian users. Non-vegetarians face other issues when it comes to food consumption when related to vegetarians and hence it is important to address their issues too.

If you want to completely detoxify at home, purchase the book. You will get loads of good advice and information.

Using Natural Herbs For Detox

For the body to function well, it is important to clear the accumulated toxins. In order to regain energy, the body needs to be healed. Body detoxification or body detox using herbs is one way of clearing unwanted toxins from the body. However, it is not a single step but a series of steps forming a process that ensures that the body's natural ability is supported for dispelling toxins effectively everyday.

Along with herbs there is another way of cleansing the body of toxins that enter it. Restricting or stopping the consumption of products such as refined sugar, alcohol, carreine, drugs, tobacco, household chemicals, synthetic or petroleum based paraphernalia is an excellent method of detoxification. Instead of these products start eating natural organic diet foods, get regular exercise and drink sufficient amount of water to facilitate the body detox process. It is easy for the body to adjust to a gradual change that is better when compared to other procedures.

The herbs listed below have been known for years to be effective as home remedy.

· Psylliumhusksandseedscontainahighcontentoffiberthatgentlyfunctionsasa natural laxative. It can be used after soaking its seeds in water. Generally, psyllim is considered to be adaptogenic that supports healthy bowel functions. It can also be used in treating irritable bowel diseases like diarrhea. Its gelatinous substance absorbs toxins after soaking and hence is popularly used for body detoxification.

· Gravelroot(Joepyeweed)andHydrangearoothelpindissolving,expellingand preventing crystals and stones in the kidneys and bladder. It is necessary to ensure that your kidneys are free from any obstructions that can affect the good working condition that is required for the elimination of toxins.

· Cascarasagradaisalsousedasanaturallaxative.Ithelpsinstrengtheningthecolon muscles and is safe even when used for a longer duration.

· Alderbuckthorn'sbarkisanothersubstanceusedbutitnecessarytofirstdryitandstore it for a year at least as the fresh barks are too strong and can be toxic.

Body Detox Made Easy!

- Juniper berries promote the overall health of the urinary system. It strengthens and detoxifies the urinary tract, kidneys and the bladder. It is an excellent cleanser but should not be used for a prolonged period of time as it can cause overtaxing in the kidneys.

- Nettle helps in detoxification and has properties that apply to more than just the urinary system. However over use of nettle can display the same effects as juniper berries.

- Burdock roots and seeds have similar properties as nettle. It has cleansing and mild diuretic properties but also has stronger effects. Burdock can help in the removal of heavy metals in the body.

- Cypress, celery, basil, lemon, rosemary, fennel, patchouli and thyme contain oils that are essential for the effective flushing of toxins that are present under the skin. They also stimulate circulation of the lymph.

- Milk thistle and dandelion root help in strengthening and cleansing the liver. Silymarin, which is present in milk thistle, helps in not only protecting ht liver but also in its regeneration. Waste products present in the kidneys and gallbladder are removed by dandelion root.

There are numerous ways of body detoxification at home. You can avail the benefit of natural remedies by using these wonderful herbs. Feel good about rejuvenating yourself.

Procedures For Natural Body Detox

It is not easy to set up a detox or cleansing program. There are various procedures that you need to undergo. These procedures include physical examination, health history examination, mineral level tests, dietary analysis, biochemistry tests and other related tests in order to diagnose your complete health status. All these tests can help in assessing the appropriate natural procedures that you should follow to clean your body up.

Note that analyzing your current health status, symptoms and diseases related to your lifestyle, inherent or familial patterns and your diets can help you create a detox plan for your body which best suits you.

You must remember that every healing procedure necessitates a plan that should be followed through in order to get good results.

1. Good Diet. People who lack nutrients and energy require a diet that has high nutrients and proteins to improve the health. Fatigue, low functioning of organs and mineral deficiencies should have a diet that supports it. However sometimes it becomes necessary to clean your body for a couple of days to eliminate old debris. It also helps prepare the body for building new and healthier blocks. if different stresses, travel and food are congesting you, eat lightly and drink juices for a couple of days. It can make a difference. You should also eat foods that are high in carbohydrates, low protein foods and foods that are vegetarian for a few days. Mild detox consists of vegetable meals that add proteins required in the body. A lot of vegetables along with fresh fish also help in energizing the body.

2. Utilizing natural herbs. Different organs of the body have a tendency to develop high levels of toxins. Colon is one such organ. Always remember that the large intestine can accumulate a lot of toxicity that can result in the organ functioning sluggishly. Therefore, different detox programs have been developed as a solution to this problem. A cleansing diet consisting of fiber supplements help in cleaning and toning the colon. These supplements include acidophilus culture, aloe Vera powder and betonite clay. Enemas using diluted coffee, herbs and water can be utilized for cleaning the liver.

3. Regular exercise. Exercise helps in stimulating sweat that in turn helps in eliminating toxic wastes through the skin. It also improves the general metabolism of the body and aids in the overall detoxification of the body. Regular aerobic exercise helps maintain a non-toxic body as this prevents bad habits. However, excessive exercise leads to an increase in toxic productions in the body and therefore exercise must be associated with adequate fluids, minerals, vitamins and antioxidant replenishments and other detox related principles.

4. Regular bathing. Cleaning of the skin and accumulated toxins is very essential. Saunas and sweats are often used for body purification using enhanced skin elimination. It is suggested that before bathing everybody should dry brush the skin at least once.

5. Massage therapy. It helps in supporting detox programs. Also it helps in stimulating body eliminations and functions and promoting relaxation that helps clear tensions, mental stresses and worries.

6. Resting, relaxing and recharging. This is an important part of the rejuvenation process. It helps the body and mind rebalance. Practicing regular yoga is a powerful exercise that helps in regulating the breathing and also in obtaining an active and balanced aura.

Choose the procedure that cleans your body correctly. It makes you healthier and therefore happier.

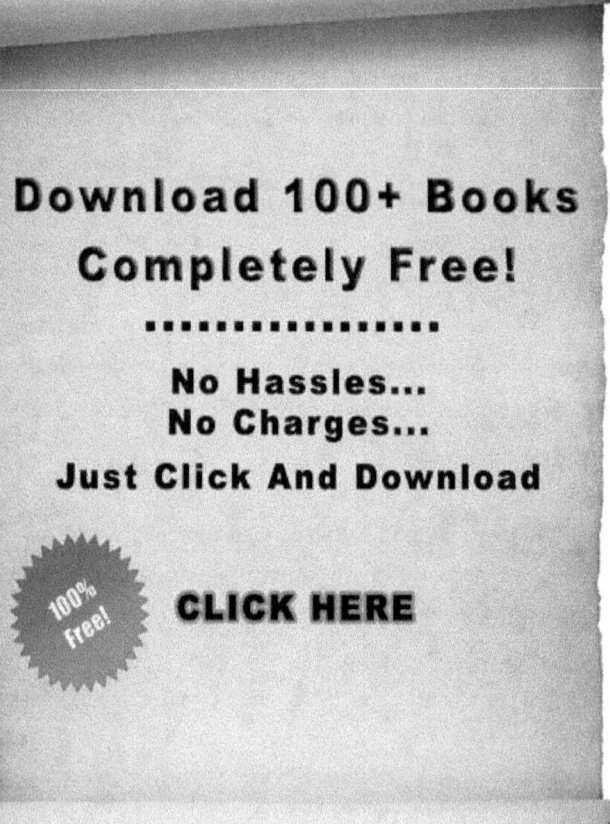

This Product Is Brought To You By

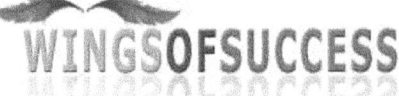

www.ingramcontent.com/pod-product-compliance
Lightning Source LLC
LaVergne TN
LVHW021054100526
838202LV00083B/5910